Schizophrenia

An Essential Guide to Overcoming
Schizophrenia

*(The Coping With Psychosis and
Schizophrenia Self Help Handbook)*

Sharon Johnson

Published By **Jackson Denver**

Sharon Johnson

All Rights Reserved

Schizophrenia: An Essential Guide to Overcoming Schizophrenia (The Coping With Psychosis and Schizophrenia Self Help Handbook)

ISBN   978-1-77485-527-0

No part of this guidebook shall be reproduced in any form without permission in writing from the publisher except in the case of brief quotations embodied in critical articles or reviews.

Legal & Disclaimer

The information contained in this ebook is not designed to replace or take the place of any form of medicine or professional medical advice. The information in this ebook has been provided for educational & entertainment purposes only.

The information contained in this book has been compiled from sources deemed reliable, and it is accurate to the best of the Author's knowledge; however, the Author cannot guarantee its accuracy and validity and cannot be held liable for any errors or omissions. Changes are periodically made to this book. You must consult your doctor or get professional medical advice before using any of the suggested remedies, techniques, or information in this book.

Upon using the information contained in this book, you agree to hold harmless the Author from and against any damages, costs, and expenses, including any legal fees potentially resulting from the application of any of the information provided by this guide. This disclaimer applies to any damages or injury caused by the use and application, whether directly or indirectly, of any advice or information presented, whether for breach of contract, tort, negligence, personal injury, criminal intent, or under any other cause of action.

Table of contents

Introduction

Schizophrenia is an extremely serious mental illness that affects people. Numerous studies have revealed that the condition is recognized in almost every single society in the world regardless of the fact that the local manifestations differ and its symptoms are somewhat "culture-bound'. The most common time for it to manifest is at the end of teenage years and can be extremely distressing for the sufferer and their family members as well. There is no one-stop solution All orthodox psychiatric treatments recognize that a combination of mental, social and medical approach is needed.

However, it is among the most poorly recognized conditions. Despite the fact that there are some excellent books available that explain the condition to general public - like those produced through the Royal College of Psychiatrists - textbooks are written by professionals. It is difficult to locate the most concise description of what the condition is, what's known about it, and the treatment options for it.

The book aims to fill the void. I'm sure it won't be able to do it well and I will keep an eye on feedback , and in the event that I've missed important aspects, I will attempt to rectify these in future versions. The book was written by an UK psychiatrist (using an pseudonym) but it is written for anyone around the globe although some references to NHS practices will not transferable to other countries.

Chapter 1: Schizophrenia

Around one-in-200 of people who live in the U.S. will strengthen schizophrenia throughout their lives. Anyone has the potential to contract this illness. Schizophrenia can manifest in a variety of unique ways and may manifest in a variety of unique ways.

Schizophrenia is a serious cognitive illness that affects people who interpret reality differently. Schizophrenia can also with a variety of delusions, hallucinations and incredibly disordered questions and behavior that can affect day-to-day everyday functioning and may be debilitating.

Patients with schizophrenia require continuous treatment. The early treatment can also help detect signs of schizophrenia prior to the onset of serious illness and could also improve the long-term perspective.

How can I define schizophrenia?

Schizophrenia is an intellectual illness, which is known by the term "psychosis."

Psychosis is a mental condition in which an individual cannot distinguish what is real from what's imagined. Sometimes, people suffering from psychotic disorders lose touch with reality. The world may also seem like a maze of confusing images, thoughts and sounds.

How common is schizophrenia?

Schizophrenia is more prevalent than many people think. Around one out of 200 people living in the United States will improve schizophrenia throughout their lives. It's also crucial to realize that schizophrenia is a condition with many distinct symptoms and may manifest in a variety of different ways.

Schizophrenia is not similar to schizophrenia is not the same as "split character." A split personality is a different type of intellectual disorder. Split personas are much less common than schizophrenia.

Who is afflicted with schizophrenia?

Anyone can get schizophrenia. For males, signs of psychosis typically begin in teens or in the 20s. For women, signs of psychosis and symptoms typically begin around the age of 20 and 30s.A individual is no longer considered to be a sufferer of schizophrenia until the signs and symptoms persist for at the least of six months.

What exactly is "paranoid schizophrenia?""

Paranoid schizophrenia is a type of schizophrenia. In this kind of schizophrenia the individual's false opinions are generally about being targeted or punished by someone. The individual could be able to listen to the voice of anyone who they believe that they are being punished. The person may also accept as factual the belief that they have been chosen specifically to fulfill an unidentified mission. These are only some examples of the possible false beliefs that an individual suffering from this illness could also be prone to.

Other forms of schizophrenia comprise with "catatonic" schizophrenia as well as "disorganized" schizophrenia. Different forms of schizophrenia could be characterized by same symptoms.

Signs and symptoms

Schizophrenia can cause problems with questioning (cognition) behavior, as well as emotions. The signs and symptoms may differ, but typically, they are accompanied by hallucinations, delusions or speech that is disorganized and a diminished ability to function. Some symptoms may include:

*Delusions. These are false notions that are no longer founded on the reality. You might think that you're being attacked or even slapped with a slap; certain gestures or comments are directed towards you; your potential is extraordinary or the world is watching you; everybody else has fallen in love with your or that a major catastrophe is about to happen. Delusions can be seen in the majority of people suffering from schizophrenia.

*Hallucinations. They typically involve hearing or seeing things that aren't there. However, for those with schizophrenia, they are under the full weight and an effect on daily experience. Hallucinations may occur at any level of the senses but hearing voices is the most common hallucination.

*Disorganized questioning (speech). Inferred disorganizedness from the speech that is not organized. Effective communication can be impeded, and the answers to questions could be totally or in part completely unrelated. Sometimes, speech may comprise putting together meaningless phrases which aren't comprehended, but are known as a phrase salad.

Very disorganized or bizarre motor behaviors. This can manifest in various ways, ranging from childlike playfulness to erratic anger. It's not always about an end goal, which is why it can be difficult to complete things. The behavior can include the inability to follow instructions, an inappropriate or odd postures or posture, an inability to response, or vain or inappropriate movements.

*Negative symptoms. This is a sign of a diminished or no capacity to behave normally. For instance, a person may overlook hygiene issues or display a lack of emotions (doesn't look at the camera and doesn't change facial expressions or speak in monotone). In addition, the individual may also be less enthusiastic about every everyday activities, and socially withdraw or fail to experience pleasure.

The signs and symptoms may vary in their nature and severity with time with periods of worsening and disappearance of symptoms. Certain signs may also be present.

For men, symptoms and signs usually start in the early or mid 20s. For women, symptoms and signs typically begin around the end of their 20s. It's not common for children to be identified with schizophrenia , but it is uncommon for those who are older than 45.

The signs in teens

The signs of schizophrenia seen in adolescents are similar to those seen for adults, however, it can be more difficult to identify. It is also possible to be in this section due to the fact that the initial symptoms and signs of schizophrenia in adolescents are typical for normal improvements throughout the teenage years, for example:

*Withdrawal from friends and family.

A decrease in overall school performance

*Trouble sleeping

*Irritability, depression or depressed mood

Lack of motivation

Additionally, recreational use of substances like methamphetamines, marijuana, or LSD occasionally some time cause similar symptoms and signs.

In comparison to schizophrenia signs and symptoms among adults, teenagers could be:

* It is possible to believe in delusions.

*More likely to experience hallucinations that are visible

When should you see a doctor?

The majority of people with schizophrenia are unaware that their problems originate from an intellectual condition that demands medical care. Therefore, it is often the responsibility of family or friends to offer assistance for those suffering from schizophrenia.

Assistance to anyone who may be suffering from schizophrenia.

If you think that a person that you have observed may be showing symptoms of schizophrenia, talk with them regarding your worries. While you shouldn't pressure anyone to seek specialist help, you may offer support and encouragement in helping your loved one in finding a licensed physician or an intellectual fitness specialist.

If you feel your loved one is posing the risk of harming themselves or others, or does not provide his or her own food and shelter may consider calling 911 or other emergency responders to assist them to ensure that your loved person can be assessed an expert in intellectual fitness.

In some instances hospitalization in emergency situations may be necessary. Involuntary commitment laws to intellectual fitness treatment vary through the state. Contact local companies for intellectual fitness or police departments within your area for more information.

Suicidal thoughts and behaviors

Suicidal behavior and thoughts is common among human beings suffering from schizophrenia. If you are a loved one who is at danger of taking their own life or has attempted suicide attempt, be sure that anyone stays with them. Contact 911 or your local emergency number immediately. If you think that you are able to do this in a safe manner, transport the patient to the nearest emergency room.

The Reasons

It's not yet clear what causes schizophrenia, however scientists believe that a combination of genes, intelligence chemistry and environment can contribute to the amelioration of the condition.

The problems that are caused by positive naturally occurring intelligence chemicals, which include neurotransmitters, such as glutamate and dopamine may also contribute to schizophrenia. Neuroimaging studies show differences in the Genius form and central fearful machine of humans suffering from schizophrenia. Although scientists can't be certain of the importance the changes they observe, they insist the fact that schizophrenia can be a condition that can be characterized as a talent disorder.

Risk factors

Although the precise cause of schizophrenia isn't known however, certain elements seem to enhance the risk of causing or triggering schizophrenia, such as:

*Having a family history of schizophrenia

*Some pregnant women may experience problems, such as the inability to eat or exposure to viruses or toxins that could also have an impact on the development of talent

*Intake mental-altering (psychoactive or psychotropic) capsules through the teenage years and into young adulthood.

Complications

If left untreated, schizophrenia could lead to extreme problems which affect all aspects of our lives. Other issues that schizophrenia can cause or be connected to are:

*Suicide, suicide attempts and thoughts of suicide

Anxiety and anxiety-related disorders and Obessive Compulsive Disorder (OCD)

*Depression

Alcohol or other drugs, including nicotine

*Unability to work or go to school

*Homelessness and financial issues

*Social isolation

*Health and scientific concerns and health

*Being victimized

Agressive behavior, even though it is not common

Prevention

There is no method to prevent schizophrenia, however , sticking to the prescribed method can help prevent the recurrence or aggravation of the symptoms. Researchers also believe that learning more about the risk factors for schizophrenia may result in earlier analysis and treatment.

How can schizophrenia be diagnosed?

If there are signs the doctor is likely to conduct a full medical record and a physical examination. While there aren't any laboratory tests to diagnose schizophrenia, your physician will probably use a range of diagnostic tests -- for instance, MRI and CT scans, or blood tests to rule out a physical illness as the cause of the symptoms.

If a medical professional determines no medical reason to the symptoms he/she may recommend the patient to a psychologist or psychiatrist or healthcare professionals with specialized training in diagnosing and treating intellectual disorders. Psychologists and psychiatrists utilize specially made equipment for evaluation and interview to determine if a person is suffering from schizophrenia. The medical professional or therapist base their analysis on the individual's report of symptoms and their observations of the person's mental state and behavior.

The therapist or health professional decides whether the person's symptoms point to a specific disease as described within the Diagnostic and Statistical Manual of Mental Disorders (DSM-5), that is published by the American Psychiatric Association and is the most popular reference book for diagnosing intellectual disorders. According to DSM-5 the diagnosis of schizophrenia is conducted if an individual exhibits two or more fundamental symptoms, the first of which is hallucinations, delusions or a speech disorder for at least a month. The various core symptoms are extreme disorganization and a decrease in emotional expression. Other DSM-5 guidelines for an analysis of schizophrenia are:

*The level of work, interpersonal families, or self-care is significantly lower than what it was prior to the onset of symptoms.

*An indication of disturbance that has been present for at least six months.

*Schizoaffective disorder and depressive bipolar disorder with psychotic symptoms are largely ruled by psychotic signs.

*The disorder has been eliminated. caused by drug abuse or any other medical condition.

Treatment

Schizophrenia needs to be treated for the rest of your life, even after symptoms and signs have diminished. Treatment with medications and psychosocial remedies can help manage the symptoms. In some instances hospitalization is also required.

A psychiatrist experienced in treating schizophrenia usually provides treatment. The team of treatment could include a psychologist as well as a social worker, psychiatrist nurse, or even an individual case manager to oversee treatment. The full-team method could work in clinics with expertise in schizophrenia treatment.

Medicines

Medicines are the mainstay of treatment for schizophrenia, and antipsychotic medications are the most frequently prescribed medications. They're used to manage symptoms and signs of altering the neurotransmitter intelligence dopamine.

The purpose of treating antipsychotic medications is to alter symptoms and signs as well as symptoms to the most minimal dose. The psychiatrist can also consider unique drugs, extreme doses or combinations in time to achieve the desired result. Other medications could be helpful with depression, for instance antidepressants or anti-anxiety medications. It may take several weeks to notice an improvement in the symptoms.

Since the use of medication for schizophrenia may cause serious adverse side effects, those suffering from schizophrenia might be hesitant to take the drugs. Inability to cooperate with treatment can also impact on the drug selection. For instance, someone who has a difficult time taking medication for a long time may also want to receive injections instead of taking the pill.

Consult your physician regarding the advantages and effects of any medication prescribed.

Second-generation antipsychotics
Second-generation, more recent medical drugs are generally sought-after due to the fact that they offer a lesser chance of serious side effects as opposed to first-generation antipsychotics. Second-generation antipsychotics comprise:

*Aripiprazole (Abilify)

*Asenapine (Saphris)

*Brexpiprazole (Rexulti)

*Cariprazine (Vraylar)

*Clozapine (Clozaril, Versacloz)

*Iloperidone (Fanapt)

*Lurasidone (Latuda)

*Olanzapine (Zyprexa)

*Paliperidone (Invega)

*Quetiapine (Seroquel)

*Risperidone (Risperdal)

*Ziprasidone (Geodon)

First-generation antipsychotics
First-generation antipsychotics can cause typical and possibly significant neurological effects, including the possibility of causing an ailment of motion (tardive dyskinesia) that may be unable to

be irreversible. First-generation antipsychotics consist of:

*Chlorpromazine

*Fluphenazine

*Haloperidol

*Perphenazine

They are generally cheaper than antipsychotics of second generation especially the commonly used varieties, which are an important when you require a long-term treatment.

Long-acting, injectable antipsychotics

Certain antipsychotics can also be administered as an intramuscular or subcutaneous injection. They are generally given every and every two to four weeks, depending on the medicine. Consult your physician for the latest information regarding injectable drugs. This could be an option if you have the desire to use smaller doses of capsules. It could also help with adhering.

Common medications that are in stock as injections are:

*Aripiprazole (Abilify Maintena, Aristada)

*Fluphenazine decanoate

*Haloperidol decanoate
*Paliperidone (Invega Sustenna, Invega Trinza)
*Risperidone (Risperdal Consta, Perseris)

Psychosocial interventions
After the psychosis is gone and you are able to continue with medication as well as social and psychological (psychosocial) intervention are essential. They could also include:
*Individual therapy. Psychotherapy could also aid in normalize thought patterns. Additionally, learning ways to handle stress and to recognize early warning signs of relapse could help people who suffer from schizophrenia to manage their condition.
*Social competencies training. The focus is on improving the social interaction and verbal exchange and increasing the ability to participate in everyday activities.
*Family therapy. This provides assistance and education for families with schizophrenia.

*Vocational rehabilitation, supported employment and. It focuses on helping individuals with schizophrenia who are able to discover and keep jobs.

The majority of people with schizophrenia need some form of daily home help. A lot of communities offer programs that assist people with schizophrenia in finding work and housing, self-help business and in disaster situations. The case manager or member of the team will be able to help locate the resources. With the right treatment, many people suffering from schizophrenia are able to manage their condition.

Hospitalization

In the event of a disaster or of severe illness hospitalization is crucial to ensure security and proper nutrition, as well as plenty of rest and hygiene.

Electroconvulsive therapy

For those suffering from schizophrenia and who do not respond to treatment Electroconvulsive therapy (ECT) could be thought of. ECT is also beneficial to those who suffers from depression.

Helping to cope and providing support

Being a person with an intellectual illness such like schizophrenia could be a challenge both for the individual or woman who suffers from the condition as well as for family members and friends. Here are some ways to deal with the situation:

*Learn about schizophrenia. Knowledge about the disease could aid the person suffering from schizophrenia to realize the importance of adhering to the treatment plan. It can also help family members and family members to understand the condition and show more compassion to the person who suffers from it.

Keep your focus on the goals. managing schizophrenia is an ongoing process. Keep in mind your therapy goals will help the person or woman suffering from schizophrenia to remain focused. Let your loved one know the responsibility of controlling the illness and pursuing the goals.

Avoid drinking and using drugs. Consuming nicotine, alcohol, or recreational medications could make it difficult to treat schizophrenia. If you have a loved one who is dependent, quitting could be a real difficult task. Find advice from the fitness and health care team on the best approach to take to address this problem.

Ask about social offering assistance. These programs could be in a position assist with housing costs transport, and other day to day activities.

Learn to manage stress and leisure. The person with schizophrenia and their loved ones can benefit from strategies to reduce stress, such as yoga, meditation or tai-chi.

*Join a assist group. Support groups for humans suffering from schizophrenia may help those with schizophrenia connect with others suffering from similar issues. Support organizations can also aid family and friends in dealing with the challenges.

Chapter 2: The Symptoms That Can Confirm Schizophrenia

According to ICD-10 the concept of a complex of symptoms is being created which requires different criteria to be met in order to identify schizophrenia. In this scenario positive or negative ones are differentiated.

Positive symptoms can take forms of behavioral characteristics such as hallucinations, delusions, hallucinations and delusions that are beyond the normal behavior of people.

Negative symptomatics are characterized by deficiencies in the way people behave in comparison to healthy individuals. They include flat-tensive affective symptoms (severe diminution of emotional interactions with other people, insanity tranquility, unintentional emotional reactions) as well as a lack of interest, social withdrawal as well as inattention to personal health. A disorder called I is common to people affected. The main distinctive about this is that the lines between our egos and outside world are considered to be permeable. Additionally, one's own self as well as the body, thoughts and thoughts, along with the surroundings are seen as being a little strange. The patient is a part of an actual world and an euphoric world. It is becoming increasingly a clone from the world. The diagnosis is founded on the following symptoms:

1. Echo of thoughts, ideas and inspirations thoughts that draw attention broadcasting

2. control mania, influence delusion, causing feelings perceived your body thoughts, actions, or sensations and sensations of mania

3. Voices that comment or slide-logically sound

4. Persistent, culturally inappropriate , or absurd belief

5. Persistent hallucinations in every sense mode

6. Tears from thoughts or thoughts and become a flow of thoughts

7. Catatonic symptoms include Arousal, postural stereotypes stupor, or negativism.

8. Negative signs, such as obvious Apathy, speech perception unbalanced or flattened affects.

A prerequisite for the diagnosis of schizophrenia is at minimum the presence of a distinct symptom from the groups one to four or at least two signs of groups 5 to 8. These symptoms should have been nearly all the time during more than a month. In the initial diagnosis, a thorough physical as well as neurological examination should be performed. To determine the differential diagnosis, examinations of blood and liver values as well as kidney values and brain function are required. There are also conditions that exhibit similar symptoms like physically justified psychoses such as social-affective or affective disorders, and borderline disorder. These disorders must be considered prior to the diagnosis of schizophrenia is made. [Fussnote 3]

Subtypes and forms of schizophrenia

Kan distinguishes paranoid schizophrenia, catatonic schizophrenia, hebephrenic schizophrenia, residual schizophrenia, and schizophrenia simplex.

It is the most frequent type. It is characterised by persistent hallucinations and paranoid delusions and mood swings (irritability and anger, fear, and distrust) and disturbances in thought (distortions of thought processes or absurd word rewriting abruptly consuming thoughts, sudden thinking that is not rational).

In the cases of catatonic schizophrenia these disorders of the brain are often the primary subject of. There is a change between extremes, for example, the state of arousal or stupor (reduction of the response to the environment , and changes in behavior, such as silence, for a longer duration) as well as between commands automatisms (automatic conformity to instructions) or negativism (resistance to commands or attempts to change into). There are also physical compulsions or compulsions and absence of movement and motor restlessness. In this type of condition there are verbal perseverations in the form of the utterances of a language are usually repeated in the same manner and are often interpreted as to be meaningless.

Affective disorders are a common occurrence as well as impotence and disruptions in thinking are the hallmarks of schizophrenia known as hebephrenic. The drive and determination disappear There is no objective and there is no plan. The person affected behaves recklessly and in a way that is unpredictable. The mood is dull and incongruous, caused by laughter, grimacing or hypochondriac complains, as well as repeated expressions. Thoughts are erratic, speech is disorganized and unclear. The sufferers are often isolated.

The recurrence of schizophrenia is often accompanied by deficiency in drive and affective poverty, as well as social withdrawal.

A form that is symptom-free is schizophrenia simplex. The psychotic process is slow and the symptoms that are productive are not present. The typical symptoms of schizophrenia are not fully developed, and the progression is moving, sometimes over many years.

Hallucination and Manic

Delusions and hallucinations are the most striking and common manifestations of schizophrenia and they need to be discussed in greater detail.

Hallucinations are believed to be perceptions , without similar stimulus source and, consequently, are perceived as senses that can be considered to be real perception of a sense. Acoustic hallucinations are experienced by half in patients. Visual hallucinations are are in 15 percent and haptic hallucinations occur in 5percent. The most commonly reported auditory hallucinations can be described as "voicing". Certain types are so typical of schizophrenia that a diagnosis as per ICD-10 may be made immediately. They include dialogical voices where the patient is able to hear voices that are in the form of speaking and then counterspeech (as other people talk about him or in his presence). Comments are heard in every day treatments. The person in question wears a new outfit and then a voice comments (often in a derogatory way) on the procedure "Now you can change your clothes". Imperative voices offer instructions, for instance, the voice instructs the person who is concerned "go into the lounge and switch on the television". Imperative voices are danger if the person in question cannot separate himself from them. For for example, they give directions that can lead to criminal charges. Alongside the auditory hallucinations you can also experience optical hallucinations which are quite uncommon. The person experiencing the hallucinations does not observe everyday or extremely bizarre images, not-existent people animal, objects, or complicated scenes. Patients provide examples of "aerial images of the desert" or "a rodent tail that emerges from their buttocks". Through haptic or tactile hallucinations can be described as perceptions where the patient is influenced or altered by or within the body, either magnetically or electrically through rays, devices, as well as other physical phenomena. The reason for this is false beliefs based on inaccurate beliefs about the external world. Delusion is seen in 90% of patients in its course during their condition. The person who is affected relates the actions of others to themselves. These tend to involve persecution and ideas about relationships where the real-life situation of the individual concerned is not recognized. Manic content can refer to areas of impairment due to poisoning or persecution, hypochondriac fears, great ideas that are expressed in the form of unique talents or abilities, or even a religious and political motivations. [Fussnote 4]

Chapter 3: What Happens When An Affected Person Feels About The Disease

People who suffer from the condition often feel as being healthy. The symptoms such as delusions or hallucinations are believed to be real , and the environment they live in is able to convince them that they are sick. There is often an absence of disease for those who suffer. The reason for the decline in performance is often blamed by the medication or work environment. However, there are those who are sick and at the very least, have an inkling that something isn't right in their lives. They can come up with strategies for assistance to help them deal with their mental illness and stay clear of excessive stimulation. For instance, they've developed a way of assessing the point at which it is too noisy or chaotic for them and then resign themselves. There are many sufferers who seek to ease themselves by drinking alcohol. They feel the effects of drinking alcohol to help them ease their stress, relax and get along with others more quickly. It also increases the chance of suicide among people affected[Fussnote 5.

The daily life of the psychiatric hospital is a study conducted by Erving Goffman

Erving Goffman Erving Goffman, an Canadian sociologist, examined the life of a psychiatrist clinic through research, and revealed what differentiates them from the patients and what they can expect out of their patients. The main idea can be said to mean that "the most significant factor that makes a person the patient is not his condition however, it is the institution which he is at mercy of" (Goffman 1972). The characteristics of institutions in the following way They are a counter-cosmos to the normal world of social interaction and are models constructed by the society themselves. The life that a patient has is an expression of the life that of those who would be considered to be the "normal" individual. Goffman is able to distinguish between the preclinical phase as well as the clinical and post-clinical phases.

The psychiatric evaluation of a person is only significance from a sociological perspective standpoint, as it alters his social situation. This alteration of his destiny happens after he's sent to a rehabilitation and nursing home. As a result, all individuals belong to this group, and was somehow able to get into the system of a psychiatric hospital.

There are different types and severity of the illness that psychiatrists experience with him , and in relation to the traits of the layman who exhibit it.

The commonalities of patients with psychiatric disorders have been explained in the work of Goffman as the assignment of an identity and destiny shared by the society. It is an ongoing social change process, triggered through the struggle with the similarity of conditions in psychotherapy clinic and the formation of psychodynamic groups by former patients that are an attempt to create a safe community in a community.

The sociological observer believes that the insanity or unhealthy behavior, a result of the social disconnection of the observer from the person's condition and the social environment, is not a result of the mental illness or illness of the individual. He is convinced that he's in an environment that isn't any different from other communities he's studied.

"Voluntary Patient "voluntary patient" makes up a small portion of patients in preclinical care. These patients with mental illness are admitted to the clinic due to their own beliefs and beliefs, which is good for them. The starting point is experiences with the "threat of self". The symptoms are then identified in this instance and the new details about one's self are hid from the world. If someone chooses to visit an institution that treats patients the relief could result in to an increase in the condition as it could be confirmed objectively, which was prior to that a an individual experience.

In his research, Goffman mainly examines patients who have voluntarily entered the psychiatric hospital which is the case for the majority of people.

Patients visit the hospital due to the fact that they have been repressed by their families or were threatened with a crime or under duress by police escorts or under false beliefs, that were intentionally sparked by other people (especially for young individuals). The exclusion model here is the idea that the patient is deprived of his connections and a substantial part of his rights from the beginning of their hospitalization. Moral issues are expressed in the form of feelings of loss, fidelity and bitterness
The social start of the professional career of the preclinical patient is different from

the psychological beginnings of the illness. The case histories of mental illness reveal the violation of conditions of immediate coexistence. For instance, in the home and at work in semi-public institutions such as churches, and in public spaces such as parks and streets. The person who is at fault is deemed to be a 'transgressor' for these offenses However, not all violations result in being hospitalized. Other consequences of admission to an psychiatric hospital include e.g. exile, divorce, detention or loss of employment or expropriation of property of property, outpatient psychiatric treatment etc. Goffman believes that a variety of other psychiatric effects could have occurred for patients who are hospitalized in the opposite direction, resulting in numerous violations leading to a successful complaint. Similar instances occurred, but remained ineffective. What are the features of hospitalization for patients with psychiatric disorders?

The thesis reads: "The official concept of society is that the inmates of mental hospitals are there primarily because they were born. The argument can be summarized as:" The official concept of society is that patients of psychiatric institutions are there due to the fact that they are mentally ill. But, in the event that the "mentally sick" outside of clinics exceed the number inside the clinics, it is possible to suggest that those suffering from mental illness do not result from the mental illnesses, they suffer rather from luck. "(Goffman, 1972). Goffman is able to determine this by examining social-cultural status, the glaring of transgressions and their proximity to a psychiatric hospital as well as the range of treatment options available. However, to the degree that the number of "mentally sick" in the absence of clinics is greater than patients who are in clinics one could argue that people with mental illnesses do not result from mental illness, but rather from luck. "(Goffman, 1972). Goffman is among the career-related incidents that can be a result of socio-economic status, the public visibility of transgressions, closeness to a psychiatric facility and the range of treatment options.

Agents contribute on the journey from the status of a citizen to that for the person who is suffering. The most trusted friend is typically the closest relative who provides support during moments of crisis. They are expecting to be left behind during times of crisis, and also expected to rescue him from the dreadful fate that is waiting for him.

The patient is the one who appears to trigger the pathway of the preclinical patient to the clinic. He is an employee, neighbour, employer, family member or doctor, police officer social worker, teacher lawyer, cleric etc. In the group of complainants, there are professionals legally authorized to conduct the briefings, referred to as mediators. If the preclinical is now an actual patient in the clinic, then the deciding actor is now the clinic's administrator. The next friend is put in the role of the accountable person by making appointments in the clinic prior to when they are scheduled and then urging the preclinical patient to be aware of these. The patient is then left with the impression that his next friend becomes an ally of the specialist , and that he is becoming more and more into a patient. The patient is able to sense that an unwelcome alliance is being forged in his favor by both his most trusted confidant as well as the expert. Moral experiences are marked by a sense of bitterness, rejection and/or deceit.

In the perspective of the patient the chain of relevant numbers functions as a type of funnel for fraud. Every step of the process from the individual to patient results in a decrease in the standing of an adult. Every agent involved attempts to conceal the truth. As the chain is slowly transferred from the patient to the medical facility in the future, the patient will be aware that his health was compromised and the peace of all involved parties is kept. This is a moral reality that is a further barrier to the world outside during the time of the incident.

The mediators of the transition from the citizen to that of the patient are interested in having a second trusted person to act to act as an advisor or protector for the patient. The patient's confidant could take on the care and affairs of the patient that is otherwise a burden for the clinic. In the same way that a patient becomes an individual, the person who is a confidant will be transformed into an advocate via the intermediaries.

The result to the person receiving treatment is that the person is requesting for assistance and protection from dangers could be authorized by the administration of the clinic. This means that he has the impression that the small size of the relationship doesn't suggest anything about the reliability of the individual. The intermediaries' chains often determine the status of the closest confidant by ensuring the patient that hospitalization is the best option.

The person confiding in is then liberated from the feeling of guilt toward the patient as an ethical obligation for the mediator was offered to him. The next person who is familiar with him will then assume crucial roles for mediators and the clinical administrators. They could, in turn, perform important roles for the patient. The main stage in the career of the preclinical patient is realisation of the society that was ejected as well as his future fellow human beings.

At the start of hospitalization, the patient attempts to stay completely alone and refrain from talking with anyone. He tries to stay off any contact or involvement in the scene, and to observe what others think of him. In addition, the visiter's inability to talk to the patient, or the absence that follows the visitor's visit. However, relatively quickly the patient with psychiatric issues is able to be anonymous and is able to take part in the normal social interactions within the hospital community. He has a tendency to stay in the hospital to the side, for instance, when encounters in the clinic of a person who whom he has known from the past. So, he is able to discover his way through the structure of the station and this change in the way he behaves at the start of the hospital stay . It is described by the hospital staff as the ease of access for the patient, and the initiation into the world of. The patient experiences moral humiliation or extreme changes in living conditions, such as restrictions on mobility and living in the community, the diffuse authority of many people, disobedience resulting in the loss of rights, etc.

The patient is instructed in the psychiatric hospital that the deprivations and limitations which he is experiencing are part of his treatment needs and treatment which in turn reflect the present state of himself. The admission of a patient to a specific area within the facility is portrayed as a sign of the overall social purpose of his position as an individual.

The station system demonstrates how the physical environment of an institution can be utilized to alter the perception that people project about themselves. In extreme situations an image of a mental illness is presented to the patient. It states that the entire history was a self-inflicted loss and that if one is to be considered a serious person for who he is, then his behavior towards individuals, as well as his self-image , will change once someone is at a certain stage in his career, he creates an image of his life. It is composed of present, past and the future. This abstracts, chooses, and alters the events to ensure that his current circumstances are seen positively. The perception of the person in question causes him to adjust his defense to the basic values of society. Goffman describes an apologetic self-presentation. It is an argument that defends one's beliefs as well as one's personal beliefs.

The patient is seeking motives and explanations for his hospitalization. He tries to prove a tragic story to prove that he's not suffering from illness and that the problems the patient has faced have not resulted in other people suffering, his resume was worthy and the hospital wrongly assigns him the status of mind.

The inmates interact in the clinic and have different the reasons behind their confinement. Based on the lies told by one another, a full social function within the patient community could be created. These are typical social functions of the information network . They are people of similar status and serve in the capacity of an audience stories that support one's self.

The hospital staff have the benefit in examining the patient's past. The patient is deemed as a failure, and the claims he makes about himself are fabricated. The difficulties that the patient is causing are inextricably linked to his personal version of what he's doing. If his version of the truth is scrutinized by medical professionals, this aids in ensuring that the patient is willing to collaborate.

The case history helps demonstrate that the patient is suffering and in what degree it was appropriate to send him to go to the clinic. A listing of events that were symptomatic could have been an outline of the entire CV. Examples include actions that are far-reaching where the patient was unable to exercise judgement. Furthermore, the conditions which a layperson might describe as unclean, impure or childish, etc. They are not.

The report might also contain details that the patient posed in response to embarrassing questions, and that was presented as contradictory claims to the facts. Goffman states that not all levels of staff are able to handle the psychiatric diagnoses of the case report without moral neutrality, and instead, they respond in a manner that is more informal to such issues regardless of the manner in which they respond, even with gestures and tone during the interactions between the patient and staff as well as in the gathering of the staff member with whom the patient may be present. In certain hospital settings, the access to reports of cases is reserved to doctors and higher ranks but the lower levels of nurses also are able to access the informal or second-hand data. Additionally, regular medical record is available to all levels of staff and contain the same information as the data recorded in the case report. The patient is frightened because he is confident that the information relevant to him are collected correctly and that he has no control at all on the people who take the information into consideration, and therefore, he experiences the dissecting impact of the report.

Communication patterns, both formal and informal, of hospital staff enhance the impact of the report. The negative actions of patients in a specific segment of the hospital's population will be observed by those who oversee other aspects of his life at the clinic. In the discussion with staff, personnel members are able to discuss their thoughts regarding the patient before deciding their future treatment and attitudes. The patient then gets the impression that there is a plot to harm the patient, even though this is done with the intention of doing his benefit. On a casual level the recent actions of the patient during lunch are discussed by staff members via an informal chat. In hospitals, this details about the patient are shared, and the patient would prefer to keep private. The information is utilized by medical staff in different grades to challenge the claims of the patient.

For instance, questions are addressed to him during the diagnosis. He is required to give false answers to avoid having to be viewed as a failure in self-esteem and the right answer is provided to him. If the patient goes to a physician or nurse to ask for more privileges or to request his release, he is confronted with a question that is not a valid answer without recalling an unjust act committed by the patient.

In particular, in the beginning of his hospitalization It is often difficult for patients to develop a sense of self as he is exposed to continuous changes. He shifts departments and stations often, which means that he alters his life both to his advantage as well as to his disadvantage. Every one of these changes results in an abrupt change in their living environment and is similar to the rise and fall from one social group to another. Additionally, his fellow patients who he is able to identify in a certain degree, change their lives - and the patient himself gets an impression of change in society regardless of whether he does not feel it directly his own. The psychiatric facility is viewed as a rehabilitation facility for patients who have moral results. If the patient realizes and accepts the absence, he may use this as an opportunity to live an appropriate life, and ask the staff to assist in the effort with kindness or privileges, and tolerating.

Once a patient is able to endure situations where he continuously is at risk of being exposed and may be considered a threat or rejected but without the power to influence the situation and thus take an important step towards socialization. The past and present developments are being constantly analyzed morally, which results in an exceptional form of adaptation that cannot be described as an ethical form of self-images. When a patient discovers that personnel and other patients are able to are able to take on and diminish them in a way that is not terribly revealing, and realizes that the self image is something that can be swiftly created, destroyed and rebuilt. Ultimately, one learns that it's capable of being a self no matter the treatment options that the clinic may offer or deny. When this happens the process of building up and dissolving the self becomes a humiliating game. The person experiences that he is not an army, but an open, small city. the society reveals a real self. Goffman states that the Heilanstanstalt creates a type of cosmopolitan wisdom and an inability to think about the bourgeois status one's self. [Fussnote 6]

Chapter 4: Epidemiology, Illness Course And

explanation models

Schizophrenia is a common affliction across the globe in equal numbers. The risk for life, that is the likelihood of having a person with schizophrenia throughout his or her lifespan, is around one percent. In Germany and other Western European countries about 0.5 to 1percent of the population is affected by the illness. In Germany it means that around 800,000 people are affected the disease. It is referred to as a new disease incidence of 2 to 4 instances per year, and 10,000 people.

Men living in Germany are affected 3 to 5 years before (between the ages between 15 to 25,) more than females. In general, females are more susceptible to the disease.

The most common disease occurs between the ages of 25 and 34 of age.

When you reach 14 years of age around 2% of people are affected. The most common time for the disease is between puberty and the 30th-35th year of life. After around 40 years old, one is a victim of schizophrenia that is late and, as of 60, one is diagnosed of schizophrenia in the elderly.

10 % to 12 percent of the patients are able to remain for a 15 - year time frame without presenting any further symptoms. 43% have chronic symptoms are observed. 82% of the patients suffer a relapse within 5 years. 10 % - 15% of patients die following a suicide and the rate of suicide is greater than 30 times over the entire population.

The course of illness

Prior to the onset of the disease, in three-thirds of cases, from a week to one year-long stage, which is also known as a prodromal period is observed. In this stage, non-typical symptoms, like social withdrawal and depressive moods can result in a bizarre behaviour. When you enter the psychotic acute stage, the most severe symptoms of the illness develop. The phase is characterised through psychotic episodes. Following this phase, which can be accompanied by a number of episodes or a persistent symptoms of recovery could occur, or be unaffected.

Resorption symptoms are seen in around 50 percent of cases. In one third of patients, the condition is nearly completely disappeared. In some cases, the productive-schizophrenic symptoms remain chronic in about one-third of those affected. This results in diminished social skills and hospitalization. It's not possible for patients to live their lives independently. They have to be taken care of in residential homes or monitored communities, or permanently confined in a medical clinic. There is a possibility of healing or a spontaneous improvement in the later stages of chronic schizophrenia is feasible. Many sufferers aren't able to manage their daily life regardless of whether the psychotic impulse has disappeared. Postremissive disorders can be a possibility with depressive moods as well as anxiety disorders Exhaustion states. In general, a prolonged prodromal stage, stress, an insufficient intelligence level and a delay in the start of treatment may affect the future development. [Fussnote 7]

Explanation models

There isn't a single cause of schizophrenia. The root cause of the disorder is a multifactorial structure of the conditional of psychological, biological and social elements. It is known as the Vulnerability-Stress Model. functioning model of schizophreniathat considers the multifactorial nature of schizophrenia and is the most commonly used model to explain the illness.

In addition, genetic factors are also of a significant importance. Research has proven, that if you fall ill, with a increasing degree of connection, the risk, which is also associated with schizophrenia rises. Based on twin studies as well as adoption studies, the proportional risk of the illness. If both parents are suffering from schizophrenia, there is a chance of developing the illness for the child. The risk is 40 percent. If a parent is down ill, the risk is at 10 percent. If twins are twinned, there is the chance for having a twin fall ill too, with a range of 10 to 15% and for identical twins, with 50 percentage.

Normal siblings are born with a rate of 10 percent. Half-siblings, niecesand nephews and grandparents with a likelihood of around 3percent. Studies on adolescents of T. Kohler (2005) reveal a 10-20 percentage chance of disability for children with schizophrenia-related parents regardless of whether they are in the same household as parents or teenagers who aren't affected. The risk for children with parents who do not suffer from schizophrenia doesn't increase when they reach the age of when they have diseased adoptive parents. Additionally, there are biochemical explanation studies, which are founded on the dopamine hypothesis.

One can speak of an inherited metabolic disorder. This is a result of an over-sensitiveness of dopamine receptors within certain brain regions. Additionally, structural characteristics in the brains of people suffering from schizophrenia were discovered in accordance with neuroanatomical findings. Although psychosocial factors aren't confirmed by research, but they are believed to affect how the illness. Psychogenic factors are:
I-Deficits (I-weakness and brittle ego-boundaries) Communication issues (constantly inconstantly contradictory information provided to children) issues with the roll assignment (child serving as a replacement partner) and premorbid personality characteristics (Contactability vulnerable) and the possibility of stress-inducing or traumatizing life situations.

The model of stress and vulnerability was developed in the work of Zubin as well as Spring in 1977. It supposes that congenital elements interact with environmental influences which can trigger a schizophrenic illness. Vulnerability is also known as "thin-skinnedness" (also known as "vulnerability" and is a reference to the possibility of being susceptible to a illness. Certain hereditary disorders are at the root of a certain psychological vulnerability. To trigger this specific stress (stress) has to be added that is not overtaken by the person who is vulnerable. Stress may be a defensible life occasion (death exam, death loss of employment marriage or pregnancy,) or a tangible and potentially lasting strain. Adaptability refers to the ability of an individual to adjust effectively to stressful situation (coping methods). If vulnerabilities are triggered by stress and the ability to adapt of the human being becomes disrupted, schizophrenia can be seen. [Fussnote 8]

Chapter 5: Therapy

To treat schizophrenia, a multidimensional treatment method is suggested. In the initial stages of illness it is essential to undergo inpatient therapy following the cessation of symptoms of psychosis, outpatient treatment is suggested. The treatment is usually combined medically and psychotherapeutically. Additionally, various psychosocial strategies, such as day-care for outpatients and counseling are included.

The basic treatment is usually psychopharmaceuticals. In the initial phase of general therapeutic objectives obviously, the objectives are at the point of acute. This includes the establishment that the relationship between therapeutic and patient clarification of the illness and treatment strategies removal and reduction of illness in self- and external danger, integration of family members, referees and other participants, reduction of social effects and motivation to self-help.

The post-acute stabilization stage should follow by implementation of rehabilitation strategies. Also , in this stage, an established therapeutic relationship is essential. Treatment of social and cognitive impairments and other symptoms of negative nature are addressed. The patient is encouraged to take self-help measures. Awareness of the disease and active participation are encouraged. In this stage, a more thorough explanation of disease and treatments is required. Regarding education and prevention of relapses and involvement in the family members and other people of reference is possible if the people involved are in agreement. Individual strategies for coping are created and conflicts within the family and in the community are analyzed to reconcile. The support is provided to improve the stability and increase the number of social connections and rehabilitation strategies are developed or shared with. [Fussnote 9]

Pharmacotherapy

Psychopharmaceutical-therapy is used particularly in acute disease phases. The focus here is on antidepressants, neuroleptics and tranquilizers (for instance and Valium). Neuroleptics are used to treat psychotic symptoms like hallucinations and delusions. Neuroleptics are extremely effective in the reduction of positive symptoms. It is important to distinguish between high-potent middle-pinned, non-doped, and middle-pin neuroleptics. They naturally, do not come without adverse negative effects. But, pharmacotherapy isn't to be discussed further because it is too large a portion of medical therapy.

Psychotherapy

Psychotherapy is a method of helping, through the use of conversations with the client and the therapist specially trained to assist the patient is able to manage emotional and psychological issues. There are many kinds of psychotherapy. They differ in the goals as well as intensity, duration and theoretical foundation.

In the process of designing psychotherapy, it's essential to cater to the demands and needs of the affected as well as their families and shape the therapy offerings to meet them. It is crucial that the therapists you choose to work with have the appropriate training and experience in the treatment of ill patients.

In what is known as "supportive psychotherapy "the patient is actively involved during the course of treatment for their illness. In particular, he gets information on his illness as well as treatment options, and also the factors that are impaired. In turn, the motivation to treat the patient is increased. The patient's life and medical issues are discussed, and possible solutions and options can be discussed.
Behavioral therapy can help reduce cognitive impairments and enhance social

abilities. With the patient, for instance, strategies to distract can be developed that help him manage different symptoms of his illness. Additionally, it is recommended to implement the family therapy programs, which give the family members support in dealing with the disease. Important elements of psychotherapy are also the symptom management, training of social skills and everyday skills, stress prevention and stress management, addressing family problems and the overcoming the incomprehension of the surroundings[Fussnote 10]

Sociotherapy

Socio-therapy is a way to enhance the potential and social abilities that the client. It is not akin to psychotherapy or pharmacotherapy, geared towards the surrounding environment of the person being treated. They include occupational therapy and work-related therapies, as well as rehabilitative measures like rehabilitation centers or residential groups, long-term vocational rehabilitation as well as accommodation in workshops for disabled people. These elements are crucial elements in the treatment of schizophrenics.

Partially inpatient treatment programs like clinics for night and daytime hours also are part of this category. This is why it is intended to create the conditions that aid in the development of the abilities needed by the people affected to live independently and to be able to integrate into society.

It is essential to be attentive to both. Also, avoid the requirement for the individual affected. The process of activation, and thus the combating of the loss of interest, the absence of motivation and the day-to-day structuring should be gradual and be in tune with the requirements of the person affected.

It is also essential to connect with others slowly so that you can get rid of the solitary state. Through activities that are shared in the group, such as social contact as well as daytime structure and exercise can be carried out. Families and other relatives should be mindful to adapt their style of communication to the particular situation of the person in question. A highly emotional approach to communication can cause stress for the person affected and may cause him to become overwhelmed. If family members are uncertain about this, it's advisable to consult with experts within the context of psychotherapy.

Aid to institutions

The physician is the initial contact point for the person who is concerned. He will provide the required initial treatment. If there are any signs of abnormalities and the patient is referred to a neurologist who is a resident or a psychiatric facility.

Medical psychiatrists typically provide the treatment with regular visits and medications. If the treatment fails the psychiatrist may be able to refer his patient into a psychiatric institution. It is essential to ensure that the neurologist is accessible for additional treatment after discharge from a hospital for psychiatric patients. Should the patient be not willing to undergo further treatment and prefers to continue treatment by his physician at home it is possible for him.

The psychiatric hospital is usually thought of only when the patient is located close to the facility. Certain psychiatric hospitals also include a clinic ambulance that performs the same functions as the nerve surgeon. For treatment at a stationary location, a variety of methods of treatment are appropriate. The psychiatric university clinics typically have very few beds, and generally treat patients who have an initial-line disorder. The psychiatric specialty hospitals are typically huge and are situated in an idyllic location. These hospitals offer the broadest and most differentiated therapies available.

Also, there exist psychiatric units within general hospitals. The benefit is that close co-operation with other departments is feasible that is essential when mental illness is linked with physical illnesses.

There are private clinics that provide mental therapies. The treatment is not covered through health insurance, and private hospitals, patients are typically treated for in light instances.

All types of institutional support are concerned with the treatment which is voluntary by the patient. Patients have the right to end treatment at any point and then leave the hospital at any time. However, there is the possibility of compulsory admission which is only permitted in hospitals specifically approved which have stations closed. The mandatory instruction is controlled in accordance with national laws. These compulsions can be imposed when a patient puts at risk his health or life or the wellbeing of others and the risk can be avoided with other methods. In all cases there has to be a diagnosis of the mental disorder and then a decision has to be taken as to whether a mandatory directive should be issued.

Apart from inpatient and outpatient treatment facilities in addition, there are various treatment alternatives. There are counseling facilities, that can be accessed to offer the individual seeking aid and also for their family members who wish to be educated or educated. Particularly in teenagers the difficulty is to discern whether the symptoms are normal puberty signs. Counseling centers can be helpful in these instances.

In the middle of outpatient and inpatient treatments, there are partial stationary therapies, which take the form of night and day clinics. In a day clinic patients are usually working from morning until afternoon. Talks with individuals or in groups are held, medical treatments are offered along with group activities and leisure activities. Clinics during the day give patients the structure of the daily routine that is crucial for patients. Clinics at night are mostly employed for rehabilitation in professional settings. Patients stay in the evenings and at night in the clinic, and during the day, he is at go to work (possibly part-time or at a facility for people with disabilities). It is also possible to speak with caregivers and receive medical treatment. On weekends, patients are able to be at home or in the clinic.

If you live at home, psychiatry services for socially isolated people can be a source of assistance. The services are typically provided through social or social worker. A regular discussion is held between the client and the social worker. Psychological support plays a vital role in this. Patients require a trustworthy person, and someone who is able to understand and can support them. They also aid with administrative processes and doctor's appointments. The majority of the work is done in collaboration with psychiatrists and the psychiatric clinics.

There are legal rules which require that a care worker receives a caregiver in the event that he becomes capable of handling the care of his own affairs on his own. (Care laws – SSSS 1896 - 2008 Civil Code, Federal Republic of Germany). Caregivers provide care to provide care in the areas of medical treatment financial matters, as well as the issue of the where the patient lives. Family members may seek assistance from the qualified magistrates or the notary. As a guardian, family members or other people may be appointed.

In addition the obvious help through friends or group self-help. It is essential to tailor the various therapeutic methods and their individual combinations to the particular symptomology of the patient, while considering the capabilities and preferences of each patient. [Fussnote 11]

Chapter 6: The Psychosocial Treatment And Rehabilitation

Rehabilitation is a crucial part of treating schizophrenia sufferers. When a clinical diagnosis is made based on ICD-10, and the disease symptoms of schizophrenia are evident there are a variety of treatments to be considered. Psychotherapy and dependency on psychopathology is the initial step, being followed by psychoeducation, assisting psychotherapy , and working with relatives.

Psychoeducation is the process of transferring relevant information about diseases and treatments to the affected person and their family members. Furthermore an analysis of problematic areas must be conducted. Problems with these areas can impact persisting symptoms as well as social skills and cognitive capabilities. However, issues with family interactions may also be present. If these areas of disturbance have been identified, a variety of options can be implemented. Family intervention can be helpful in the treatment of family-related disorders. The main components of these interventions are behavior analysis, communication training methods for problem solving, as well as techniques for coping with specific problems.

If you are experiencing difficulties in social skills If you are experiencing difficulties with social skills "social skill development" is recommended, through which social skills are taught. This includes conversational skills as well as professional rehabilitation, household and housing management and management of medication as well as leisure and recreation Self-care and personal hygiene using public transport food preparation, and management of money and public authorities.

Rehabilitation encompasses vocational rehabilitation, medical rehabilitation,

occupational integration, as well as long-term treatment
job opportunities in the particular job market.

Cognitive rehabilitation is recommended when cognitive impairment is present. Skills for interpersonal problem-solving such as verbal communication, social perception are crucial.

To facilitate dealing with the signs of illness, coping strategies need to be developed. On one hand, they are disability-coping and symptom-controlling strategies for coping. On the other hand, specific coping strategies for managing the illness (sensitization for specific reactions to stressful events). Rehabilitation programs aim to being largely integrated into work, but however, they also aim for social stabilization. Naturally, everything is dependent on the severity of disability caused by disease. Rehabilitative options that may be considered are gradual increases in the hours of work per day, or occupational integration working from a part-time station, accommodations in a workplace for disabled persons, outpatient day care centers as well as assisted living. [Fussnote 12]

Community-based help systems that integrate into the community are a different component of rehabilitation. This is the term used to describe team-based or community-based care systems. They are seen from nurses, psychiatrists as well as psychologists, social workers, and Ergotherapists. They could aid in the coordination and cooperation of patients suffering from schizophrenia. They can also help with the continuous therapy process and help reduce hospitalization. Outpatient, semi-stationary and stationary aids are all part of this category and have been described.

Another crucial aspect of rehabilitation is structures for rehabilitation and promotion. For instance, in the case of those who are in the workforce in the first place, the psychosocial specialist of the primary posts should be turned on during inpatient treatment to ensure that the workplace is maintained on the first job market. To help with the professional rehabilitation of individuals who suffer from schizophrenia and want to go back to work, programs that provide rapid employment promotion must be implemented and designed based in a workplace, as well as supporting trainings. If you are unable to live on their own and require assistance in finding suitable housing suitable for those who are unable to live independently. Groups of self-help and rehab programs following an acute stage are crucial assistance in the reintegration of those suffering from schizophrenia.

Studies on the social environments of schizophrenics

If one studies research into the social networks of people with schizophrenia It is apparent that there aren't many studies on the marital or life partners of sufferers.

It is most likely that people suffering from this condition have a difficult time forming steady relationships or aren't necessarily linked to their partners. The majority of studies focus focused on family research. In this article an overview of different studies regarding the social network that patients have will be utilized to study the topic to be studied in the field.

Jungbauer conducted a study on schizophrenia patients' partners between March 1999 to May 2000. He conducted 49 interviews in narrative format of which he carried out 28 interviews for an extensive analysis of the case. His aim was to discover the way that life partners and spouses of the patients feel about the day-to-day relationship. The initial point of departure was the subjective quality of the couples. The selection of students was conducted through inpatient, semi-stationary, and outpatient mental institutions. The couples were married and unmarried interviewed, who reside with the patients in a household that is shared.

In the next section, a few of the findings of research will be discussed.

The average age of all the sample is 46 years old. Seventy-three percent have a spouse who is the sick partner , and 75% have children who are joint. The interview included 28 male and 24 female couples were interviewed. Of them two-thirds of the respondents were skilled workers 10% were self-employed, and 8 percent of them were students. The time of the survey , there were 42 percent, with 17% of them unemployed and 6% of them were at the age of retirement. When the survey, those who were interviewed have been in a relationship with their partner for approximately 15 years or in a steady relationship. For 44% of instances, the partner became in the course of schizophrenia at first in the course of their partnership as well as the condition was present within 56% of cases. 87 percent of the affected partners were receiving regular outpatient therapy when they took part in the study as well as 19%

participants themselves suffered from mental illness.

The findings were presented as a conciseand condensed format. The study revealed that psychotic crisis in patients may cause an extreme stress on the patient's partner. There's a sense of shock, despair and anxiety in the early stages of the illness. The beginning of the illness is perceived as abrupt shocking and overwhelming like a crisis. The patient is seen as radically confused, strange, and frightening. The person is suspicious, aggressive and terrified. The family members are unable to control their emotions in precisely the reason they understand that at the start of the illness , almost not much about the illness or the potential aids.

In the event that the person is placed in a psychiatryfacility, both partners will experience what is known as "clinical shock". Hospitalization inpatients can be an extensive cut on the normal day of relationship. Suicide attempts by patients are also possible in this stage, and can may have a negative impact.

If the illness is already present before the formation of a relationship it is possible that the psychological effects of crisis, which are commonly felt, are usually identical to an experience that is firsthand. The problem is less stressful when the partner is a person who has experienced mental illness.

If there is an indefinite course of disease, the gradual onset of the disease can cause other stressors. It is perceived as a gradual process of creeping and the environment in the family and in the relationship is disjointed and angry and communication is reduced. The absence of "clear" signs (such like hallucinations) is also a challenge for the spouse to understand the changes as mental illness. In the later stages of the illness, acute stress may also be experienced, particularly in the event of repeated psychotic episodes. However, these stressors are considered to be less severe than when they first began the illness because the people affected are more informed about the symptoms of schizophrenia and opportunities for assistance. But, the patients have set their own limits to their possibilities to get relief, which can be another burden.

The vast knowledge of the disease and the learned coping strategies are not enough to protect you from the fear of new assaults. Stress accumulation leads to a significant decline in the individual's quality of life and also the well-being of the partner. Partners feel isolated and overwhelmed by family and other tasks that need to complete.

Many of the partners also complain about the unwillingness to work with doctors and the introduction of treatment. The patients who are affected are not that they are being taken seriously. Doctors are accused of a lack of dedication and indifference.

Stress and tensions that arise in the daily relationship can be evident during the psychotic relapses, as well as during the phase of symptom-free. They are, so to say, ongoing stresses on partners. The negative effects of medication, symptoms and behavioral issues are also evident outside of psychotic relapses. This causes radical changes in the couple's relationship as well as the family's day-to-day life.

If the patient becoming retired or otherwise, the patient's partner will have an entirely different perspective on life as well as a different life circumstance and changes in their roles.

A lot of partners are extremely stressed because of their intense awareness of the signs they're announcing. The risk of conflict in the family is significantly enhanced, not the least due to the emotional instability as well as the constant appearance of the sufferer in their home. A lot of partners suffer from the loss of their mental well-being and experience depression and exhaustion. The social network is becoming shrinking and becoming less.

The team will devise a variety of strategies for coping. Through providing members with information about schizophrenia, they develop an essential skill to deal with and counteracting the loss control. The argument
Family support services as well as crisis management, and a peaceful, disease-focused lifestyle are among the likely ways to cope for the couple. The assessment of the disease and focusing on the things positive about the couple's relationships are available as cognitive and emotional strategies for coping. To reduce the risk of incurring charges, couples dedicate themselves to routine recreation, increase their commitment to work and when necessary, make an opportunity to relocate.

The majority of patients experience the illness as a deep cut in their biographical history and attempt to categorize the condition into their own personal history. The definition of relationship and the common sense perspective are in the process of being questioned.

Many couples feel obligated to remain with their sick spouse and see a possible separation is a violation of current values.

In general, a lot of emphasis is put on one's own family and life and serious feelings ofthe top.

On the contrary, a positive health condition, family engagement of the partner and a traditional conception of marriage and partnerships, positive assessment of one's personal coping capabilities as well as a long-term shared life and a general positive relationship of balance may have an effect of stabilization. [Fussnote 13]

There are a variety of research areas that are part of schizophrenia research. One of them is "Expressed Emotion Research. "Expressed research on Emotions" is concerned with the relationships among family environment and relapses in patients suffering from psychotic schizophrenia. "It is now clear that the way families deal with each other is vital to the development of schizophrenia" (Johannes Jungbauer 2005, The Partner of Schizophrenic patients in the treatment of schizophrenia, p. 21).

The idea that is "Expressed Emotional Research" was devised by the research group that was formed around George W. Brown. In 1962, Brown and his colleagues demonstrated their first-ever study that atmosphere of emotion in the family is a significant indicator of the outcome of patients with schizophrenia. In their study they carried out an interview known as the "Camberwell family interview (CFI)" in which they interviewed the significant family members. The interview was focused on the mental health of the loved one. The risk of relapse has been identified for those who returned following treatment in families that have an excessive amount of emotional involvement than people with low involvement in social life. This finding has been confirmed multiple times. It should be noted that the index of "Expressed emotion" was constructed through the interview process, and from an evaluation of the severity of the patient's antagonistic enmities, the amount of negative comments about him, as well as the level of emotional involvement. In addition, para-verbal signals were included. It was believed that the behavior displayed during the interview could be observed in daily situations. [Fussnote 14]

Angelmayer (1995) includes diverse research findings regarding social networks for schizophrenics. This means that their networks are smaller than those of healthy people or people suffering from other mental disorders, and the percentage in family members large. The relationships they have with their families are typically fragile and prone to failures. The social network of patients who have a long-term history of disease is composed of those who suffer from other mental illnesses as well as friends of patients.

in 1994 Haberfellner as well as Rittmannsberger conducted a research study and discovered that contacts of schizophrenics are considered to be sufficient by patients and 54% of these are other patients or caregivers of psychiatric illness.

Rehabilitation des Patienten, dar.

Hoening and Hamilton identified sub-jective and objective stress factors that affect people with mentally ill individuals. Stresses that are objective can be seen as negative side effects of illness , such as disruption of family life expenses, financial strain and the need for medical services. Subjective burdens define how much family members really feel overwhelmed. The causes of stress are stress and tension in the body guilt, sentiments of guilt (especially parents) anger (regarding the patients negative symptoms) concerns and fears (suicide and life planning) Responsibility and obedience. The distinction between subjective and objective aspects is still being used even today. In many studies, it was discovered that female relatives are more susceptible to tension than their male counterparts. [Fussnote 15]

Chapter 7: Schizophrenia And Its Effects In The Early Years And In Adolescence

Children and adolescents form the most affected individuals. It is difficult to diagnose schizophrenia in the early years of adolescence and childhood because schizophrenia is an under-studied field in adolescents and children's as they grow older, and the adolescent stage is associated with a myriad of problems that make it challenging to identify early-onset schizophrenia. Although schizophrenia is a rare condition among adolescents and children however, it is crucial to be aware of early signs in order to be able to begin treatment.

If the first sign of the disease is prior to reaching the age of 18 it is known as "Early Onset Schizophrenia (EOS)". For the "Very early onset Schizophrenia (VEOS)" The illness begins prior to the age of thirteen. The warning signs include changes in the nature of things like social withdrawal, a lack of motivation, strange behavior, loss of a certain age feelings of affection, and aggression.

The early detection of schizophrenia-related psychosis is essential for a good prognosis of the condition. There are numerous studies regarding the monitoring of patients who have an early onset of illness or schizophrenia with early-onset. But, they are not the right topics to discuss further as the primary main focus should be on the rehabilitation and care of adolescents and children. [Fussnote 16]

A good example of rehabilitation of adolescents and children with schizophrenia is treatment offered in the "dormitory for children and young people "Leppermuhle" located situated in Federal State Hessen, in Germany. The treatment offered in this facility will be reviewed in greater depth.

The children's dormitory and adolescents "Leppermuhle" located in Buseck located in the Federal State of Hessen in Germany is a special facility for rehabilitation of children and adolescents suffering from mental disorders, including schizophrenia. Rehabilitation refers to the post-clinical areas. The home operates in the type of follow-up care following an acute clinical treatment. The home is in close collaboration in close collaboration with Department of Child and Adolescent Psychiatry at the "Philipps University of Marburg" which offers crisis care when needed. In the course of the execution in the rehab program at this home is a 6-month schedule of assistance is made available. It is a requirement to have weekly meetings and every day exchange of knowledge between therapy professionals teachers and patients and parents, which includes their participation. Therapists are responsible for the treatment of children and adolescents as well as for counseling educators. The educators offer pedagogical support for patients. The medical services offered by clinics and doctors are offered in the form of medical treatment for the patient and the counseling provided by therapists. It is the Youth Office is involved in all of these processes. Information exchange and the making of decisions is conducted between clinicians, educators, and patients in the employment office schools, training centers, and professional training (Helmut Remschmidt and his team, 2004 Schizophrenic Disorders during Childhood and Adolescence (p. 101).

It is a multidimensional rehabilitation program that incorporates a variety of methods of transportation. The people who are targeted by the home is youngsters, children and young adults suffering from a current or more serious mental impairment who require postclinical care or rehabilitation.

In the full-stationary zone, children as young as the sixth grade are examined for signs of emotional disorders, developmental issues or brain disorders, as well as part performance issues or have hyperkynetic syndrom or autism.

Young adults and adolescents with severe neurotic disorders, psychoses and personality issues are also analyzed in this section. The group of patients within the day-time group is children between seven and twelve years who are experiencing difficulties in their social behaviour and emotional issues, as well as the development of remains, hyperactive behaviors and autistic behavior patterns.

The housing groupings of the house are inspected by teams comprising of four to five professional educational forces, in each instance as well as a house economic power and psychotherapist. There are five inside housing group and ten housing groups outside and child housing groups that are decentralised and comprise another residential tract and leisure area, and in each of them, there is only one room.

There are also monitored residential groups and personal living areas. The residential groups that are supervised belong to the third stage of the idea of living in the residential area . They are intended for young adults who are 18 and above. They are 3 to 4 rooms located in a residential structure located outside the facilities (in Giessen and Reiskirchen). The living areas are offices for the educators, who provide a regular maintenance, mostly during the afternoons and the evening time. The fourth phase of the process of self-employment is supervision of single occupancy. Young adults reside in apartments that are single and are monitored by pedagogical professionals through consultations, often each week.

In addition to these types of accommodation and care, there are also groups that cater to youngsters and children who are unable or not be cared for in regular groups. They are situated on an estate of a farm, just 15km from the house. The units for intensive care are distinguished by a very high quality of care, an integrated unit the most structured day-to day program and child and teenager psychosis.

In mother-child groups, minors as well as full-time mothers and pregnant women are cared for in a peaceful residence in the heart in "Reiskirchen". Young mothers and pregnant women are able to take part in all aspects that the house provides. In the home, there is a recognized private school that is an institution for sick children. The "Martin Lutheran School" 130 children and teens are educated within 16 groups, every of which has up to nine students in accordance with the principal of the class teacher. The degree can be obtained, or secondary school leave certificate. There is also educational support for social pedagogy in the classroom or in form of a special educational support specifically for students in primary school and their parents. Based on the pedagogical model at the institution, an inter-individual learning experience for students in classes with interdisciplinary content is expected to be guaranteed. The curriculum is based on those of public schools, and it is possible to provide specific measures of support for each student. Additionally, regular classes and project weeks are available.

Following a thorough diagnosis The treatment plan provides for the creation of an individual treatment program. Therefore, rehabilitation can be accomplished through attending at the school for nursing or social therapy or occupational therapy is a possibility by utilizing pedagogical and therapeutic accommodations as well as therapies that can be carried out in the form of psychotherapy, riding therapy or occupational therapy, as well as movements therapies. The concept of treatment in Leppermuhle is based upon several guidelines: at some moment in time, changes in the degree of demands should occur before proceeding to the next step is taken, a certain amount of demands should be controlled over a specific amount of time, provided it is managed effectively over the long-term and the patient is able to have sufficient reserves to handle the additional demands.

For an expert rehabilitation, occupational therapy is provided. As a therapy area it has the wooden workshop and a nursery. There is also an office, assembly, housekeeping and occupational therapy. The first step is occupational therapy. stage of the rehabilitation of children. Skills must be taught and practiced. These is a requirement for future professional pursuits. Young people receive an assessment every quarter following the achievement of the objectives of the therapy, they are assisted by external interventions for the rehabilitation process (vocational preparation and vocational training) together in conjunction with an employment exchange "Giessen" which is located in Germany.

A part of the overall interdisciplinary concept is psychotherapy. The practice is performed by a close partnership between the therapeutic and educational personnel in the residence unit. The medical and psychological care team is comprised of psychiatrists, psychologists, and psychotherapists.

Additional offerings of the youth and children's home include the Riding-therapy program with trained Riding-therapists and Mo-pedagogy to provide a movement therapy that is largely funded by the sport pedagogical and leisure educational offers, along with various other initiatives that are implemented regularly.

The aim of the home, workplace and social integration is realized in an interdisciplinary environment, that involves institutions both external and internal as well as people. Medical and educational specialists collaborate closely to achieve their goals in the field of mental health education and career, and social interactions and personal growth through different strategies. Children and adolescents who suffer from the illness of psychotic schizophrenia have the possibility of having a complete and positive outlook for their illness. [Fussnote 17]

Chapter 8: The Soteria Draught Is An Alternative Form Of Therapy.

Soteria is an alternative therapy for patients suffering from psychoses, specifically schizophrenia-related disorders. The word Soteria originates in Ancient Greek, and means the healing process preservation, well-being and salvation. The concept was first developed and then realized by American psychotherapist Loren Mosher. In the 1970s, he opened an institution that was akin to a community California that he referred to as"the "Soteria House". It was known as the Soteria House was an alternative treatment method that was not in the psychiatric facility. Patients who were diagnosed with a psychotic schizophrenic disorder were treated and assisted. The hospital in California was closed in the middle of 12 years due to insufficient state funding.

In 1984, the Swiss psychiatrist and researcher in schizophrenia Luc Ciompi, based on the Californian model, created the Soteria establishment in Berne. The concept that was initially proposed was later developed and further enhanced by it. The nuclear components in the Soteria concept include psychosis accompanying with involvement in active ways, the restrained administration of neuroleptic medicines and a holistic approach. According to Loren Mosher, Luc Ciompi, there are two distinct Soteria guidelines.

The location should be intimate with a focus on community, which is voluntary and local-based. There shouldn't be more than 10 beds. This includes the beds for staff members. Care is given in the Soteria house 1:1. Residents are the patients who are referred to as residents in the sense of.

The social atmosphere should be safe clean, friendly with respect, upholding, shelter, security and be friendly. A family-oriented life (replacement of the family) is a goal. In relation to the social structure, no dependency issues will be created, but the freedom of individual decision-making is to be preserved. The relationship between residents and supervisors should be developed and the flexibility of the roles played by residents and supervisors is sought to attain.

The most important thing is the shared everyday household chores. They include cooking, cleaning and making music, as well as performances, and outings. The day-to-day activities play an important role.

The supervisory team is comprised of professionally trained psychiatric professionals or members of a select group of clergy. Additionally, they may be clients who have been previously treated. Training for vocational skills, which includes supervision of the work of clients and families, should be accessible to any caregiver.

The interpersonal relationships are of vital significance for the effectiveness for the treatment program. The caregivers are hoping that they oppose the psychosis while keeping an open mind and not ideologically oriented. They aim to offer the patients the opportunity to follow up with them and assess the subjective experience of the psychosis as true. It is important to keep a clear understanding of the psychiatric language avoided when dealing with patients. There are no formal treatment options. The supervisors adjust themselves to the individual's needs and help and motivate him based on his physical condition.

There is no need to administer medicines in very small doses. The duration of stay must be adequate and can differs for each patient.

Only after a prolonged stay will relationships be formed between caretakers and residents, triggers are easily identified and the hurtful feelings are expressed and felt. Also important is the post-care of the resident. The maintenance of the relationship between individuals after dismissal is sought to. This eases the transition into "normal routine" and helps in the formation of networks.

Following the establishment of the Soteria facility in Berne (which remains in existence in the present) two facilities were set up in Germany There was the Soteria situated in Zwiefalten was established in 1999 in 1999, while the Soteria in Haar close to Munich was created in 2003. There are also psychotherapy clinics that are located in Germany which are a result of Soteria that were conceived into their ideas. There are defined standards for these elements that aren't to be explained here. A single of these Soteria facilities, which is the Munsterklinik Zwiefalten will be discussed within the next. [Fussnote 18]

The Soteria The Soteria House in the "Munsterklinik Zwiefalten" located in Germany

It is the Soteria of the Munsterklinik Zwiefalten is a place for men aged between 17 and 45 years old, who are suffering from an extreme psychotic state (according to ICD-10 F2 - "People who suffer from schizophrenia"). In addition, individuals are admitted who require an environment that can provide support following an episode of psychosis or would like to lessen or decrease their medications. Treatment for mothers and children is also feasible. The desire to treat yourself is the primary requirement.

The team is comprised of nine members, comprising nurses, health workers as well as psychologists, social pedagogues and psychiatrists. The institution's management include a psychologist with a diploma and nurses for psychiatry. The medical treatment is administered by the chief doctor.

The hospital is located within the municipality located in a separate location that is separated from the area of the clinic, and has a large, lush garden. The house is built on three levels with sheben beds. The ground floor is home to common areas, such as the kitchen and living rooms, a dining room, smoking room office, restrooms, as well as a room for mothers with a child. On the top floor are two living spaces (two double bedrooms and one of which is single). Additionally, there is a second living area that is not equipped with a radio and TV there is a spare room as well as bathrooms. The upper floor is quietest. There are two rooms as well as the so-called "soft room" that is a crucial element of the Soteria concept. The "soft room" there are just blankets, pillows, and a mattress. The walls are decorated with soothing shades. The space is designed to provide the emotional well-being of residents with a psychotic state. There is also a waiting area as well as a sanitary facility and a paint room. The flooring's staggering follows the principle that "the higherthe level, the more peaceful" since the person in the acute stage requires to be irritable and understandable, and those who are close to being released requires activation.

In Zwiefalten Three treatment phases can be distinct: acute phase, activation phase discharge, or reintegration phase. The three phases should be viewed as an "red thread". The transitions are fluid and could be of different lengths. Much attention is paid to individuality.

In the acute stage it is crucial to protect the patient from external stimuli in order to alleviate anxiety and create peace. In the acute phase are typically placed inside"the "soft area". A caretaker who is devoted to the resident and is available round all hours for the patient and stays with the resident in the room. This will naturally adapt to the individual, and attempt to determine the things that could help the resident. Empathy and trust play an important role. There is a strong emotional exchange. The integration into the daily routine occurs only when the resident isn't stressed. The current needs of the resident come first. They usually involve non-verbal requirements like massages, walking, painting or other artistic pursuits.

In the phase of activation, the person is moved into his personal space the intense psychotic experience is complete. The actual reference has to be gradually restored through regular and simple work. An ongoing and practical "lived communities" is a goal. The self-confidence and self-esteem the resident is restored and he's motivated to be accountable for himself as well as his surroundings. A lot of residents wish to exchange their experiences and experiences, which is why people who can refer them to and residents of the house are on hand. Family members as well as other reference people are able to be part of this process. The guilt and shame are addressed and eliminated. The value of additional outpatient psychotherapies is appreciated by a large number of residents and is backed from the hospital.

The reintegration or dismissal phase is all about professional and social rehabilitation. There are concrete requirements and action steps that have to be carried out by the people who live there. The process of preparing for an independent lifestyle, as well as the interactions with the world are crucial. The subjects of this phase include the requests for housing and work Contact with schools and employers potential follow-up treatments at day clinics or additional rehabilitation centers are discussed, and formulated. Furthermore precautionary measures (possibly along with family members and other reference people) are discussed and planned. In the course of the stay in Soteria appointment with psychologists and psychiatrists, or outpatient care, to receive further treatment is agreed upon. In the psychiatric hospital or ambulance facility, the follow-up services may be offered by the medical director responsible for the care as well as the supervisor responsible for the area to aid in the process of detaching, which is sometimes challenging. Former residents receive regular or unplanned visits. [Fussnote 19]

What do you think you assess the Soteria concept be evaluated from a rehabilitation-related pedagogical point from a rehabilitation pedagogical perspective? Educational aids are designed to provide assistance, stabilization, development of psychological and social resources, as well as the counselling and support for relatives. These components are incorporated into the Soteria model in collaboration with psychiatric support. This collaboration between both psychiatry and social work is a major issue in the system of care for people who suffer from mental illnesses. Soteria facilities collaborate in various areas including social workers as well as psychotherapists, curative educators, and psychiatrists. So, psychiatric services and counseling care and psychosocial assistance (as the foundation for support with rehabilitation training) are provided. The fundamentals of rehabilitation are also evident within the Soteria concept. Self-help assistance is provided and there is interaction, collaboration and communication between various disciplines, as in between caregivers as well as residents (residents).

It is the complete human being with his requirements and his life story considered. The notion of "empowerment" is that it is, in the context of rehabilitation education, an oriented resource intervention. Resources within oneself should be discovered to be able to recognize and develop. The idea that everyone has resources within him which allow him to deal with the seemingly insurmountable situation comes from this concept. It's about strengths, talents and the potential. A human who is who can't help him needs to be reinforced. The purpose of strengthening is to create the conditions necessary for the vulnerable to bring his life back "under control" his own. Within the Soteria concept it is among other things that the patient receives an optimistic follow-up. From the standpoint that of empowerment implies that patients will be informed of the possibilities to transform his circumstances positively. Patients are encouraged and supported to to participate in normal activities as well as to accept responsibility be able to reintegrate into society and professional activities. Companion, understanding, activation and assistance are the main aspects, as they are the reflections of notion of empowerment.

Chapter 9: A Process-Related Of Illness

The term schizophrenia is used to describe a "process illness'. What exactly does this mean? Simply put, it means that it's not a medical condition that can be diagnosed in one sitting'. Also you can't attend an outpatient session with a psychiatrist after having experienced some symptoms, only to be given a definitive diagnosis. The psychiatrists must observe the situation for a period of time - usually for at least six months to determine the way things play out. This is because there's an array of disorders that might appear similar on first glance. They include, in the most traditional sense, psychosis caused by drugs, but there are other disorders like stress-induced psychotic disorder and bipolar disorder.

If you reflect on what we learned from the previous chapter, it is probable that things will evolve as time passes. However , timescales are typically measured in years instead of months. It isn't unusual in the real world for patients to be treated by"working diagnoses" for several months and, even years. This isn't something to be worried over or critique this is simply the way that doctors operate. The signs, whether or not they are part of schizophrenia diagnosis typically are treated exactly the same way, typically with antipsychotic medication that we'll discuss in the next section.

In the NHS nowadays there's some dispersion - patients are taken care of by different teams, based on the situation such as e.g. outpatient, day hospital or inpatient. In addition, there is an increasing tendency to employ specialists for the initial stages of the disease - 'Early Intervention for Psychosis" partially because not every psychosis can be attributed to schizophrenia, and early intensive evaluation and treatment may help to clarify the cause.

For those who are found to be suffering from schizophrenia, the majority are treated in some kind of mental health unit that typically comprised of individuals with a range of abilities. The professions that are represented typically include as psychiatry and psychological health, mental health occupational therapy, and social work and many more specialties being employed on a sporadic basis.

However, some people may not like being assisted in this manner For these individuals, an array of methods may be required in the course of time. In the context of the community, assertive outreach groups/functions can assist people by helping them to solve various issues in their homes or by interacting with people in various informal situations.

Sometimes, this doesn't result in the desired outcome and patients must be admitted to a hospital. We'll see in the next section it isn't always something they are willing to accept. Psychologists often talk about the initial 10 years of illness as being quite chaotic. However, once they have settled, the majority of patients calm down and become easier to assist.

Positive signs

Doctors and other professionals may be susceptible to be influenced by terminology. When we speak of positive symptoms, what do we mean? In essence, these are the symptoms that are apparent and appear to be quite strange to family and friends. However, on the bright side it is the symptoms that antipsychotic medications can ameliorate (and when you're lucky remove completely). Let's look at a few at a few.

Hallucinations, defined as having an experience in the absence of stimulus can be experienced through any of the five senses. The auditory hallucinations are perhaps the most well-known. They may be second-person one person who is addressing the sufferer , or third person three or more persons discussing the person suffering. Typically (though it is not the only way) they are seen as outside of the patient's head and can be annoying, abusive or insulting. They may be linked to illusions (see the section below) and may appear to originate from different body parts, such as stomach. One specific type of auditory hallucination that is some concern . It's known as an order hallucination, in which the voices of one or more people tell the sufferer to perform a task (sometimes due to pain or penalty) and the person feels that they are somehow obligated to do this, even if it is not in line with their best judgment. It can result in various negative consequences, such as injuries to the sufferer or others.

However, hallucinations may be experienced in different senses, and they are more frequent than we previously believed. Hallucinations of the olfactory sense are possible however, when they do occur, psychiatrists typically prefer to rule out any other natural conditions that could trigger them, for instance, temporal epilepsy of the lobe. The hallucinations of the tactile are common to other disorders, such as cocaine addiction, in which an ant-like sensation under the skin (formication) is a common occurrence. The hallucinations of schizophrenia can manifest as sexual experiences - seldom are they pleasant. The hallucinations that are associated with sensations of tasting can cause people to believe their food is altered or poisoned in some way. This can be an illustration of connection between hallucinations and belief that is usually false.

It is crucial to realize that people don't always openly discuss their experiences with friends, family or professionals. Sometimes, they are only 'worked out' by watching the way people behave such as responding to "voices". Sometimes, directly asking questions is the best way to find out what is happening, however in other cases, they can only discuss the issue after recovery or even not even.

A delusion is a notion that is held with a range of certainty without any evidence. Be aware that the mainstream religions that are of any kind are excluded by this definition. In general, they are quite strange and have a lot of complex "delusional" systems. They are often 'paranoid by their nature. The literal definition of the word 'paranoid is self-referential. psychiatrists too often employ it in the informal meaning of recognizing conspiracies or plots against one due to the fact that this is common in schizophrenia. It is true that believing in something isn't necessarily an issue but in schizophrenia, it can become an overwhelming concern for many individuals and causes an enormous disruption to daily life. For instance, those believing that the aliens emit harmful radiation may stay in their home and could wear aluminum foil on their heads if they dare to go out.

Another type of delusion that is common is that of grandeur. This is also a symptom frequently found in the manic stage that is a symptom of bipolar disorder. It is based on the person's past it is possible that they believe they're significant, for example, an iconic person from the past and sometimes, a religious figure or even that they are possessed by special powers or an entrusted task - usually based on their religion and beliefs. A belief that one has been chosen by God to fulfill a specific task is very typical. People with this kind of delusional faith seem to believe that they are accepted but there is a difference between the (usually rather routine) realities of their existence and the alleged consequences of their position. For instance, those who believe they are the Queen of England may not see any contradiction between their belief in this in addition to the knowledge that they reside in a bed at Rochdale (no reference to Rochdale is meant - however, we are aware that the Queen does not reside there).

Another common area of issues with schizophrenia is those that are associated with thoughts. Certain people believe that their thoughts are being implanted into their minds, and/or they are able to broadcast ideas to other people via some form of the phenomenon of telepathy. Another possibility is that other individuals can read their thoughts. This can be connected to paranoid thoughts regarding powerful individuals who control their thoughts or the society. Psychologists often use the term "formal thinking disorder". This can be a bit confusing term, better described as an illness of the way of thinking (not as the reverse of informal). There are many various ways it can manifest. In the most basic level, there's a little connection with mania, also in which it is challenging to track the course of thought during conversations. The associations are looser at this stage, while at the mid-point it is possible to discern some connection, however it is not tangential, i.e. 'Knight's move thinking'. In its most extreme form it is difficult to follow the flow of a conversation all . Unless one is able to discern the meaning of what a person is saying from the form (as psychotherapists tend to be) it can be extremely difficult to have a conversation with such a person.

The final broad subject I'm going to talk about in this article is the notion of "ideas of references". It is when a individual observes something and then draws an incorrect conclusion from it. For instance, watching a specific piece of dialogue from the soap opera and knowing it is certain that the particular dialogue was crafted specifically to convey an inscrutable message to the person. The idea in general is of drawing a specific meaning from the everyday. These ideas are deeply entangled with delusional systems to the point that one cannot anymore, perceive what an objective observer sees (or more accurately does not perceive). They may also provide you with photos that they claim to be proof of what they believe to be related to them, but regardless of the best intentions to the contrary, an impartial observer is unable to see the thing they're referring to.

Negative symptoms

It is fairly easy to diagnose schizophrenia, based on presence of several positive symptoms over a long period of time. There is also the possibility to establish an assessment of schizophrenia based only on the negative symptoms, however this is a lot more challenging as they tend to be less precise and typically show up in a subtle manner and are not noticed until in the past (or through the retrospectoscope, like doctors like to say). The majority of cases it is true that both negative and positive symptoms are present. since schizophrenia is a chronic and relapsing disease it is possible to see them fluctuate in the same way as positive signs.

One of the reasons for believing schizophrenia is a disorder with brain damage is the fact that it is very common to see an extended decline in general functioning following an 'episode' even when positive symptoms are resolving and responding to treatment. In spite of the claims made by certain drug companies, the majority of psychiatrists are skeptical of the power of drugs to alter negative symptoms. What exactly do we mean when we say?

People suffering from schizophrenia lose their inherent capabilities and abilities. It happens gradually manner and isn't necessarily apparent at first. In the case of motivation, for instance, the drive to accomplish things is lost, as is the organizational capacity to execute it.

People lose the capacity to focus, organize their finances, shop and establish relationships. The contents that they think about and the content of their conversations decreases - the phrase "poverty of thought" is often applied to this.

Negative symptoms are a major problem that the vast majority of treatment - as we will see in the next section - is focused on helping people deal with issues that arise due to their inability perform due to these. This is probably also the reason that after 10 or so years the people are less likely to leave services and more likely to seek help. Both lack the capacity to tackle issues independently and lack the desire to do so.

Medical treatment
The psychiatrist is, in the UK at the very least is often regarded as the orchestra's conductor however this has changed to a certain degree. In this sense, they have an understanding of the variety of issues that people with schizophrenia face and can

request individual colleagues who have specialist expertise to aid. But, as a doctor only the psychiatrist is qualified to prescribe medication. There can be no question that antipsychotic medicine is the only treatment which can have a significant impact on the majority of positive symptoms of schizophrenia (CBT as we'll find out below, has a prestigious function in helping with auditory hallucinations).

Today, most people will begin an oral modern antipsychotic , often called "atypicals" (to differentiate them from older antipsychotics with more side effects that were more common just a few years ago). Each drug is branded with a generic name like the olanzapine, risperidone and aripi or quetiapine. However, it could also have a 'trade name' under which it's sometimes identified. The generic name will always appear on the bottle, but. The drug can't be completely free of undesirable negative side consequences (some negative effects, such as some degree of sedation could be desired in a specific situation) and the ability of the doctor is to pair the patient to the medication and dosage that is most suitable for them. Of course, the patient who is being treated doesn't see eye-to-eye with the doctor , and this is an important aspect of psychiatry.

It is not everyone's desire to be taking pills on a daily basis and there are some who are so insecure, unreliable, or chaotic that a long-acting , injectable form (sometimes known as"depot") is the best choice (or recommended' as doctors prefer to call it). Newer drugs are beginning to be produced in this type of form, however most doctors prefer the known and tested ones that are made from older drugs to create "depots". These are typically prescribed every fortnight or monthly, depending on the kind of medication and the individual's preferences or needs.

Doses should be adjusted frequently, and often the drugitself must be altered. The majority of people have heard of NICE guidelines, and they provide that if someone doesn't respond to, or is unable to take a different drug, it is recommended to look to introducing the patient with Clozapine. It is the only drug that we can tell from evidence, is likely to succeed where other drugs have not, but it has its own "baggage" so it's worth taking the time to explain the drug.

Clozapine is among the antipsychotics that have been around for a long time. Today, it is well-known as one of the adverse effects of the so-called "typicals' (including, of course the deopt-type injections frequently used) is to reduce the amount of white blood cells (necessary to fight off infection) in blood. This is a very rare adverse effect that is so uncommon in fact that the authorities think there is no need for any specific safety net to be in place to handle the possibility of it happening. A simple monitoring and checking of the count of white cells if one is 'run down' or has a large number of infections is considered adequate.

This kind of side effect is more prevalent in clozapine which is why it was initially taken off the market. But it's such an effective medication that it was reinstated with strict safety measures that, if you consider it, has made it less dangerous than the other medications. It is manufactured by various firms and the regulations which are centrally defined apply to every. The first is that the drug must be taken from the hospital pharmacy, and is ordered by a hospital doctor (psychiatrist). Also, only a week's worth of the drug is available at a time during the first year, if not more with a strict system of blood testing set by the company that monitors the results of blood tests. This is carried out using an automated traffic light system to ensure pharmacies can only issue the drug when it is green and cannot do so if the signal is red. If the drug is amber, certain rules will be enacted by the organization that must be followed - typically, it involves testing again. In general terms, there's weekly testing that lasts for around 16 weeks, followed by weekly testing for about one year after beginning and then four weeks of testing following that. Since side effects can be reversed once you stop the medication, any serious adverse effects can be avoided.

Nowadays, psychiatrists prescribe variety of different drugs for patients suffering from schizophrenia, however these are usually prescribed to treat symptoms instead of for the primary disorder. I'll discuss some of these. Antidepressants are often required because depression associated with schizophrenia (positive manifestations) associated with schizophrenia are prevalent. Mood stabilisers can be used to regulate fluctuations in mood. Lithium can be used for increasing the number of white cells in those who dip in the amber (or even red depending on conditions) spectrum of clozapine monitoring. Anxiolytics (drugs that reduce anxiety) are frequently used, along with drugs to treat the different side effects of antipsychotics, such as stiff muscles, or'restless legs'. Some people need drugs to aid sleep (where the beneficial side effects of antipsychotics are insufficient) and some need medication to address urinary or salivatory/gastrointestinal problems associated with antipsychotic drugs.

Alternative treatment options

As I've mentioned in the previous paragraph, a wide range of people are involved in the treatment and'management of a person suffering from schizophrenia. One of the most crucial components of in the UK system is CPN/CMHN (community mental or psychiatric nurse). The job of the CPN/CMHN is extremely diverse. It includes everything from providing injections to administering formal therapy and a vast variety of supporting roles between. CPNs are typically present at home, and are the first point of call for a variety of health issues. Today, some of the CPNs' responsibilities are taken by a the care coordinator who can come from any of the various disciplines involved. The care coordinator is also accountable to develop an individual Care Plan in association with the person themselves. Sometimes this is done informal and sometimes an important meeting is held to formalize this.

Social workers as well as their assistants play a crucial part in assessing and dealing with the entire spectrum of needs for social assistance, including housing, shopping and more. Occupational therapists play a growing function in providing care, usually far more expansive than the titles they carry seem to suggest. Psychologists can assist with a variety of issues and help people overcome and confront their "voices" through a specialization of cognitive behavioral therapy (CBT). However, they are also able to assist by providing more formal counselling to address a variety of individual issues too.

Certain models of care feature flat structures where individuals from different backgrounds work together on the same task. This is typically seen in the traditional affirmative outreach model. Early intervention within psychosis teams typically place greater concentration on psychological interventions however, they do not neglect medical care.

Community treatment from a UK perspective

There have been many modifications to the way that community care is provided in the UK in recent years , and the rate of change shows no signs of slowing. In some instances, models of care are returning to their old methods - with continuity of treatment throughout, while in some cases, the fracture lines' are in a different location with one model being an initial assessment and treatment beginning 'function' that lasts some time before being transferred to a specialist team for more time care, if you require it. There's no way in a book of this kind that I could attempt to fully represent the various models being created. It is enough to say that the reality is not always as you'd think they would be. You may have to ask a basic questions in order to know what's going on with your family or that of a relative.

But what is certain to be prevalent with regards to UK UK is that healthcare is intended to be a community-based service. Sure, there are hospitals, but they have very only a few beds and you'll be fortunate to be able to stay longer than a month if you require medical attention nowadays. It's a far cry from the long-term care that was available or even fifteen years ago. There are some places that have day hospitals which you can stay at home and attend office hours. But most of them (of that there was only a handful in the beginning) are closing down because the cuts are beginning to take a bite. In certain areas, personnel will visit you for treatment, but for the majority of people nowadays they'll have to travel to community centers to receive their medical healthcare and treatments.

As we'll see later, certain people who were admitted to hospital as a'section and are now able to be released into the community with a amount of control being maintained through what is known as the Community Treatment Order (or CTO).

Legislation in England

The principal legislation that governs the treatment of those suffering from mental illness within the UK generally is a variant of the legislation is in England which is The Mental Health Act 1983. In addition, the Mental Capacity Act 2005 does have a bearing on how we deal with patients in England however, for the purpose of this chapter and limiting myself to the issues that are likely to be relevant to the majority of people who read this in England I'll stay with the mental health act's principal provisions. Before discussing the principal 'civil' procedures I'll not forget that there exists a separate set of orders that could be enacted by the courts. I will not be talking about these in the book since they won't have any effect on the majority of people.

The majority of people have heard of "being sectioned". What exactly is it? It is usually a reference to being held under

Section 2. (assessment as well as treatment up to 28 calendar days) or the section 3. (treatment of up to six months). Section 3 is able to be renewed, and there are many checks and balances that are part of the system. What is the procedure? You will find out below many people are eligible to apply for an Mental Health Act assessment (MHAA). Some people who look sick in a public space are taken care of by police under section 136 , and transported to a location of safety , usually an MH hospital, however, sometimes it is an officer's station.

The entire assessment team consists consisting of the AMHP (approved mental health professional, usually nurses, social workers or occupational therapist who is specially trained) and an accredited doctor, usually but not always psychiatrist (one with specialized training) and a doctor who is familiar with the person being evaluated - similar to their GP. The assessment is comprised of the individual along with the relative(s) being assessed, with a final determination is taken through the team about what the best way for the person to be assisted. The person that is deemed to be the 'nearest relatives' is always considered to be consulted when it is possible however, they do not have an absolute right to veto the case of a section 2, unlike when it comes to sections 3. After being'sectioned', the person must follow the direction given to them typically by ambulance, and the police might be involved when the AMHP considers it appropriate in every circumstance.

The conditions for being detained are the most important factor, which is the existence of a mental disorder that is of a kind or severity that is thought to be a reason for detention, provided there is no danger to wellbeing or security of the person or other third parties. The closest family member has the special responsibility of being able to lift the section until the clinical supervisor determines that the person poses a threat to others or themselves and there is a Tribunal must be held. Tribunal Tribunal is an independent organization under the auspices under the Ministry of Justice and all individuals who are in detention have the right to appealing both to the Tribunal and to Hospital Managers on a regular basis. They have the right to an attorney who is legally aided (where suitable) attorney to defend them. They can be assisted with an advocate.

Assistance for a loved one

I've put this chapter in due to the fact that there's an abundance of misinformation the need for help for those who seem to be mentally or physically ill and require assistance, and I'm afraid certain that some of this is due to common practice. The most common line I hear is "I cannot help someone if they wish to be assisted". This is usually a reference to the requirement that the patient attends the clinic and the family feel frustrated and in a state of despair when they try to help the family member. It is actually more subdued. The fact is that there isn't any doubt that your doctor should be the first choice of doctor. they treat the majority of mental illness. If you're concerned about a loved one, you can make an appointment with the individual's GP even if they're the same as your GP. Of course, you will not always succeed in this endeavor, but keep trying until you've tried. Another thing to remember is that doctors still make home visits , and, if they are able to explain the situation they might be able to visit someone who is reluctant or lacks the motivation to schedule or attend an appointment with a GP.

For the purpose for this section, we'll say that you failed this first line method. What should you do? You are right to ask for an MHAA on another. I'm sure you'll be taken seriously and get an answer. It is evident that this response will be contingent on several aspects, not the least of which is the family's proximity to the individual concerned. If a mother rings about a child she has witnessed getting worse over the past six months will surely receive an entirely different reaction than someone who is concerned concerning a man who has been acting oddly in the town center however both could trigger an answer. If the latter is the case you're more likely to learn what the issue is because there is no way to know.

Your next concern is how do you determine who to contact. In the daytime , all Trusts or social service departments must have some form Centralised AMHP service. If you are clear about what you need and are able to get it, you'll be directed to that department even if they're not always easily accessible via an internet search engine. In the evening, almost all local authorities have what is known as An Emergency Duty Team (EDT) to handle a variety of social emergencies, such as mental health and childcare issues which you ought to be able get an emergency number.

Make clear the issue If you are not clear, you might be urged to speak with an alternative agency, and occasionally an MHAA could be arranged. If that is the case even if the individual is not in custody, a detailed plan must be drawn up and communicated to you, in the event that you are the closest to the person or to the person in charge of their care.